# *CHOOSE PLANKING*

## *Doris A. Freema*

# Table of content

# INTRODUCTION

The history of planking as a viral trend is relatively recent, dating back to the early 2010s. The origins of the trend can be traced back to a group of Australian friends who called themselves "The Planking Team." They started planking as a way to entertain themselves and take photos in various locations, sharing them on social media.

The Planking Team's photos gained attention and quickly spread online, sparking a global phenomenon. Planking became a viral trend, with people from all around the world participating and sharing their planking photos. The trend gained further traction when celebrities and public figures began to join in, contributing to its popularity.

The appeal of planking as a viral trend came from its simplicity and the creativity involved in finding unique and often unusual places to plank. People began planning on various objects, structures, and even dangerous locations, pushing the boundaries of the trend. Some notable examples include planking on top of tall buildings, moving vehicles, or in unconventional settings.

However, while planking started as a lighthearted internet craze, it soon faced criticism and controversy. Tragically, a few incidents occurred where individuals attempted planking in unsafe environments and suffered serious injuries or even lost their lives. These incidents led to concerns about the risks associated with extreme planking and raised discussions about the responsibility of individuals participating in such trends.

As the planking trend grew in popularity, it also caught the attention of the media, leading to further debate and discussions. The trend eventually began to fade away from the mainstream, and while planking remains a popular exercise, the viral aspect of the trend has diminished over time. Despite the trend's decline, planking as an exercise continues to be practiced by many individuals as a core-strengthening workout. It is now commonly incorporated into fitness routines and exercise programs, with variations and modifications to target specific muscle groups and cater to different fitness levels. Planking's enduring popularity as an

Exercise is a testament to its effectiveness and the benefits it provides for core strength and stability.

The benefits of planking are important for several reasons: Fitness Awareness: By highlighting the benefits of planking, individuals become more aware of the positive impact this exercise can have on their overall fitness and well-being. Understanding the specific advantages of planking can motivate people to incorporate it into their exercise routines or explore it as an option for core strengthening.

Encourages Regular Practice: Knowing the benefits of planking can serve as a source of encouragement to engage in regular practice. When individuals understand how planking can improve their core strength, stability, posture, and athletic performance, they are more likely to commit to including it in their fitness regimen consistently.

Promotes Balanced Workouts: Discussing the benefits of planking helps individuals recognize its value in creating a balanced workout routine. Planking targets multiple muscle groups simultaneously, including the abdominals, back muscles, glutes, and shoulders. By highlighting these benefits, individuals can ensure they are incorporating a comprehensive range of exercises for overall fitness and muscle development. Injury Prevention: Planking, when performed correctly, helps strengthen the core muscles that support the spine and enhance overall body stability. By emphasizing these benefits, individuals can understand how planking can contribute to injury prevention, particularly in the lower back area. This knowledge encourages individuals to prioritize proper form and technique while performing planks, reducing the risk of injuries during other physical activities as well.

Functional Strength and Daily Life Benefits: Planking develops functional strength that can improve performance in various daily activities. A strong core and stabilizer muscles contribute to better posture, balance, and coordination. By discussing these benefits, individuals can appreciate how planking can enhance their overall quality of life and make daily tasks easier and more efficient.

Motivates Progression and Variations: Knowing the benefits of planking encourages individuals to explore the progression and variations of the exercise. As they become stronger and more comfortable with basic planks, individuals can

Advance to more challenging variations or increase the duration of their planking holds. Understanding the benefits motivates individuals to push their limits, continually challenging themselves and reaping greater rewards. In summary, discussing the benefits of planking is crucial to raise awareness, encouraging regular practice, promoting balanced workouts, preventing injuries, highlighting functional strength benefits, and motivating progression. By understanding these advantages, individuals can make informed decisions about incorporating planking into their fitness routines, leading to improved overall health and well-being.

# CHAPTER ONE

## Physical benefits

Planking offers several physical benefits, including Core Strength: Planking primarily targets the muscles of the core, including the rectus abdominis, transverse abdominis, oblique, and lower back muscles. These muscles work together to stabilize the spine and pelvis, promoting overall core strength. A strong core not only improves posture but also enhances performance in various physical activities.

Stability and Balance: Planking engages the deep stabilizer muscles throughout the body, including the muscles of the hips, shoulders, and scapulae. By strengthening these muscles, planking improves stability and balance, reducing the risk of falls and injuries. Enhanced stability and balance also contribute to better coordination and overall body control.

Improved Posture: As planking strengthens the core muscles, it helps support proper spinal alignment and promotes good posture. This can alleviate strain on the neck, shoulders, and lower back caused by poor posture, especially in sedentary individuals who spend long hours sitting.

Increased Flexibility: While planking primarily focuses on strength, it also stretches and elongates the muscles of the posterior chain, including the hamstrings, shoulders, and chest. This can contribute to improved flexibility over time, making daily movements and activities easier and more fluid. Full-Body Workout: Planking is a compound exercise that engages multiple muscle groups simultaneously, including the abdominals, back muscles, glutes, and shoulders. This provides a comprehensive full-body workout, promoting balanced muscle development and functional strength.

Injury Prevention: Strong core muscles and improved stability gained from planking can help prevent injuries, particularly in the lower back. By strengthening the supporting muscles, planking contributes to a more stable spine and reduces the risk of strain or discomfort during other physical activities or sports.

Metabolic Boost: Planking activates multiple muscle groups, leading to an increase in heart rate and metabolic activity. While planking itself may not be a high-intensity cardiovascular exercise, the engagement of various muscles can contribute to an overall metabolic boost and calorie expenditure.

Athletic Performance Enhancement: Planking improves core stability and overall body strength, which can translate into enhanced performance in sports and other physical activities. It can improve power transfer, balance, and coordination, making movements more efficient and controlled. Remember, the specific physical benefits experienced from planking may vary from person to person based on factors such as fitness level, duration and frequency of practice, and proper form and technique. Consulting with a fitness professional or trainer can provide personalized guidance on incorporating planking into an individual's fitness routine.

# CHAPTER TWO

# Mental benefits

Planking also offers several mental benefits: Increased Mental Resilience: Planking requires mental focus and concentration to maintain proper form and hold the position. Over time, practicing planks can improve mental resilience as individuals push through discomfort and challenge themselves to hold the position for longer durations. This mental resilience can extend beyond exercise and positively impact other areas of life where perseverance and determination are needed. Stress Reduction: Engaging in physical exercise, including planking, can help reduce stress levels. Planking provides a form of physical activity that allows individuals to divert their attention from stressors, providing a mental break and promoting a sense of calm and relaxation.

Improved Mental Clarity and Focus: During planking, individuals are required to concentrate on maintaining proper form, activating specific muscles, and controlling their breathing. This focused attention can improve mental clarity and enhance the ability to concentrate on tasks outside of exercise. Regular practice of planking may contribute to improved cognitive function and mental focus in daily life.

Boost in Self-Confidence: Progressing in planking, whether it's increasing the duration or tackling more challenging variations, can boost self-confidence. As individuals achieve their planking goals, they experience a sense of accomplishment and develop confidence in their physical abilities. This confidence can extend beyond exercise and positively impact other aspects of life.

Mind-Body Connection: Planking encourages the development of a strong mind-body connection. By consciously engaging specific muscles and maintaining proper form, individuals become more aware of their body's alignment, strength, and capabilities. This heightened mind-body connection can enhance overall body awareness, coordination, and proprioception.

Mood Enhancement: Engaging in physical exercises, such as planking, triggers the release of endorphins and other neurotransmitters associated with improved mood and a sense of well-being. Regular planking sessions can help alleviate feelings of anxiety, depression, and fatigue, promoting a more positive mental state.

Stress Management: Planking serves as an effective outlet for stress management. By engaging in physical activity and focusing on the present moment, individuals can temporarily distance themselves from stressors and reduce feelings of tension. Regular planking sessions can contribute to long-term stress management strategies and promote overall mental well-being.

It's important to note that while planking can provide mental benefits, it is not a substitute for professional mental health support. Individuals experiencing mental health concerns should consult with a qualified healthcare professional for appropriate guidance and assistance.

# CHAPTER THREE

## Health benefits

Planking offers a range of health benefits, including Improved Core Strength and Stability: Planking is renowned for its ability to strengthen the core muscles, including the abdominals, back muscles, and pelvic floor. A strong core provides stability and support to the entire body, improving posture, balance, and overall body mechanics.

Enhanced Spinal Health: Planking helps promote a healthy spine by engaging the muscles that support the spinal column. This can help alleviate or prevent back pain and reduce the risk of spinal misalignment or injuries. Increased Bone Density: Weight-bearing exercises like planking exerts a force on the bones, promoting bone density and reducing the risk of osteoporosis and fractures. Regular planking can contribute to overall bone health and help maintain a strong skeletal structure.

Improved Metabolism: Engaging in planking and other forms of exercise can boost metabolism, leading to increased calorie burning and improved energy expenditure. A higher metabolic rate can contribute to weight management and overall metabolic health. Better Digestion: The engagement of core muscles during planking can stimulate the digestive system and help improve digestion. By promoting healthy gut function, planking can contribute to better nutrient absorption and overall digestive health. Increased Flexibility and Range of Motion: While planking primarily focuses on core strength, it also stretches and elongates muscles, promoting increased flexibility and range of motion. This can improve joint mobility, reduce muscle stiffness, and enhance overall physical performance.

Enhanced Cardiovascular Health: While planking itself may not be a cardiovascular exercise, incorporating it into a comprehensive fitness routine can contribute to overall cardiovascular health. A strong core and increased muscle

Mass from regular planking can support improved circulation and cardiovascular efficiency.

Better Posture and Alignment: Planking strengthens the muscles responsible for maintaining proper posture and alignment. By improving muscle balance and reducing muscular imbalances, planking can help correct postural deviations and reduce the risk of associated pain and discomfort. Reduced Risk of Injuries: Strong core muscles and improved stability gained from planking can help prevent injuries by providing better support and protection to the body during physical activities and sports. This is particularly important for movements that involve twisting, bending, or sudden changes in direction.

Overall Functional Fitness: Planking enhances overall functional fitness by improving strength, stability, flexibility, and coordination. These factors contribute to better performance in daily activities, sports, and other physical pursuits, enhancing the overall quality of life. It's important to note that individual experiences may vary, and the health benefits of planking can depend on various factors such as frequency, duration, proper form, and individual health conditions. Consulting with a healthcare professional or fitness expert can provide personalized guidance on incorporating planking into an individual's health and fitness routine.

# CHAPTER FOUR

## Types of planks

Various types of planks target different muscle groups and provide variations in intensity. Here are some common types of planks:

Standard Plank: The standard plank is performed by placing your forearms on the ground, shoulder-width apart, and extending your legs behind you. Your body should be in a straight line from your head to your heels, and your core muscles should be engaged. Hold this position for a specific duration, gradually increasing the time as you progress.

Side Plank: The side plank targets the oblique, hip muscles, and shoulders. Start by lying on your side with one forearm on the ground, and your elbow directly beneath the shoulder. Stack your feet on top of each other or stagger them for stability. Lift your hips off the ground, maintaining a straight line from your head to your feet. Hold this position on each side for a specific duration.

Reverse Plank: The reverse plank primarily targets the posterior chain, including the glutes, hamstrings, and back muscles. Sit on the ground with your legs extended in front of you and your hands resting on the ground behind you, fingers pointing toward your feet. Lift your hips off the ground, creating a straight line from your head to your heels. Hold this position for a specific duration.

Plank with Leg Lift: This variation adds an element of balance and engages the glutes and hip muscles. Begin in a standard plank position and lift one leg off the ground while maintaining your core stability. Hold this position for a specific duration and repeat with the other leg. Plank with Arm Lift: Similar to the plank with leg lift, this variation adds balance and engages the muscles of the shoulders and upper back. Start in a standard plank position and lift one arm off the ground

While maintaining your core stability. Hold this position for a specific duration and repeat with the other arm.

Plank Jacks: Plank jacks are a dynamic variation that incorporates cardio and works for multiple muscle groups. Begin in a standard plank position and jump your legs wide apart, then jump them back together. Continue the motion, alternating the leg movement, while maintaining a stable core. High Plank: The high plank is a variation where you support your body on your hands instead of your forearms. Position your hands shoulder-width apart, directly beneath your shoulders, and extend your legs behind you. Maintain a straight line from your head to your heels, engaging your core. This variation puts more emphasis on upper body and shoulder stability. These are just a few examples of the many variations of planks that exist. You can also experiment with different combinations, such as adding leg lifts or arm lifts to side planks, to increase the challenge and engage different muscle groups. Remember to maintain proper form and technique in all plank variations to maximize their effectiveness and minimize the risk of injury.

# CHAPTER FIVE

## How to incorporate planking into your routine

To incorporate planks into your routine effectively, consider the following steps: Set Goals: Determine what you aim to achieve by incorporating planks into your routine. Whether it's strengthening your core, improving stability, or enhancing overall fitness, having specific goals will help guide your approach.

Start with Proper Form: Before progressing to more challenging variations, ensure you have mastered the correct form for basic planks. Maintain a straight line from your head to your heels, engage your core muscles, and avoid sagging or arching your back.

Determine Duration and Frequency: Decide how long you will hold each plank and how often you will include planks in your routine. Beginners may start with shorter durations, such as 20-30 seconds, and gradually increase over time. Aim for at least three planking sessions per week, allowing your muscles to recover between sessions. Warm-up: Before performing planks, warm up your body with light cardiovascular exercises, such as jogging or jumping jacks, to increase blood flow and prepare your muscles for the workout. Additionally, perform some dynamic stretches to loosen up your muscles, particularly in the shoulders, core, and hip areas.

Include Variation: To continually challenge your muscles and prevent plateauing, incorporate different plank variations into your routine. Rotate between standard planks, side planks, reverse planks, and other variations mentioned earlier. This will engage different muscle groups and provide a well-rounded workout. Progress Gradually: As you become more comfortable with basic planks, gradually increase the intensity or duration of your planks. Extend the time you hold each plank, try more advanced variations, or introduce props such as stability balls or sliders to increase difficulty. Progression should be gradual to avoid overexertion or injury. Mix with Other Exercises: Planks can be integrated into a broader workout routine.

Combine them with other strength training exercises, cardiovascular activities, or flexibility exercises to create a comprehensive workout. For example, you can alternate planks with push-ups, squats, or yoga poses to work for different muscle groups and keep your routine engaging.

If you experience pain or discomfort, modify the exercise or reduce the intensity. It's essential to strike a balance between pushing yourself and avoiding overexertion or injury. Track Your Progress: Keep a record of your planking durations and any improvements you notice over time. Tracking your progress can provide motivation and help you stay accountable to your goals. Seek Professional Guidance: If you're new to planking or have specific fitness goals or concerns, consider consulting a fitness professional or personal trainer. They can assess your form, provide personalized recommendations, and ensure you're incorporating planks effectively into your routine. Remember, consistency is key. Make planks a regular part of your routine to experience the maximum benefits. Start slowly, gradually progress, and listen to your body to create a safe and effective planking routine that aligns with your fitness goals.

# CHAPTER SIX

## Mix planks with other exercises

Mixing planks with other exercises can create a well-rounded full-body workout. Here's a sample workout routine that incorporates planks and targets, different muscle groups:

Warm-up: Start with 5-10 minutes of light cardiovascular exercises, such as jogging, jumping jacks, or skipping rope, to elevate your heart rate and warm up your muscles.

Circuit 1: Perform each exercise in this circuit with minimal rest between exercises. Rest for 1-2 minutes at the end of the circuit and repeat for a total of 2-3 rounds.

a. Plank - Hold for 35 seconds to 1 minute.

b. Squats - Perform 12-15 repetitions.

c. Push-ups - Perform 10-12 repetitions.

d. Reverse Lunges - Perform 10-12 repetitions per leg.

e. Mountain Climbers - Perform 20 repetitions (10 per leg).

Circuit 2: Perform each exercise in this circuit with minimal rest between exercises. Rest for 1-2 minutes at the end of the circuit and repeat for a total of 2-3 rounds.

a. Side Plank - Hold for 30 seconds to 1 minute on each side.

b. Dumbbell Shoulder Press - Perform 10-12 repetitions.

c. Deadlifts - Perform 10-12 repetitions.

d. Russian Twists - Perform 20 repetitions (10 per side).

e. Jumping Jacks - Perform 30 seconds to 1 minute.


Core Focus: Finish the workout with an additional core-focused exercise.


a. Plank with Knee Tucks - Assume a plank position, then alternate bringing each knee in towards your chest while maintaining a strong core. Perform 10-12 repetitions per leg.

Cool-down: Conclude the workout with 5-10 minutes of light stretching, focusing on the muscles targeted during the workout. Remember to adjust the repetitions, duration, and intensity of each exercise based on your fitness level and goals. You can also modify the exercises or add weights to increase the challenge. It's essentia to maintain proper form and listen to your body throughout the workout.

# CHAPTER SEVEN

## Recap of the benefits of planking

Physical Benefits:

Improved Core Strength and Stability.

Enhanced Spinal Health.

Increased Bone Density.

Improved Metabolism.

Better Digestion.

Increased Flexibility and Range of Motion.

Enhanced Cardiovascular Health.

Better Posture and Alignment.

Reduced Risk of Injuries.

Overall Functional Fitness.

Mental Benefits:


Increased Mental Resilience.

Stress Reduction.

Improved Mental Clarity and Focus.

Boost in Self-Confidence.

Mind-Body Connection.

Mood Enhancement.

Stress Management.

Health Benefits:

Strengthening the Core.

Improving Stability and Balance.

Supporting Spinal Health.

Boosting Bone Density.

Enhancing Metabolism.

Promoting Digestive Health.

Increasing Flexibility and Range of Motion.

Supporting Cardiovascular Fitness.

Improving Posture and Alignment.

Reducing the Risk of Injuries.

Remember that consistency and proper form are key to maximizing the benefits of planking. Gradually increase the duration and intensity of your planks over time, and listen to your body to avoid overexertion or injury. Consulting with a healthcare professional or fitness expert can provide personalized guidance based on your individual needs and goals.

# CHAPTER EIGHT

## Encouragement to try planking

Some encouragement to try planking: Challenge Yourself: Planking may seem challenging at first, but it's a great way to push your limits and see what you are capable of. Embrace the challenge and use it as an opportunity for personal growth and improvement. Efficient Workout: Planking is a time-efficient exercise that targets multiple muscle groups simultaneously. In just a few minutes a day, you can engage your core, strengthen your muscles, and improve your overall fitness. Adaptability: Planking is a versatile exercise that can be modified to suit different fitness levels and goals. Whether you're a beginner or more advanced, there are various plank variations to choose from, and progress at your own pace.

Convenience: Planks can be done virtually anywhere, without the need for special equipment or a gym membership. All you need is a small space and your body weight to perform this effective exercise.

Core Strength and Stability: Planking is renowned for its ability to strengthen the core muscles, which are vital for overall strength, stability, and good posture. By incorporating planks into your routine, you can develop a strong and stable core, enhancing your performance in other activities.

Improved Balance and Coordination: Planks engage not only your core but also the muscles in your shoulders, back, and hips. As you progress with planking, you'll notice improved balance, coordination, and body awareness, which can translate to better performance in sports and daily activities.

Mental Resilience: Planking requires mental focus and discipline to hold the position, especially when it becomes challenging. By practicing planks, you'll develop mental resilience, the ability to push through discomfort, and the confidence to overcome obstacles in other areas of life

Feel Good Factor: Engaging in regular exercise, including planking, releases endorphins and improves your overall mood. You'll experience a sense of accomplishment and satisfaction as you see progress in your planking abilities, contributing to a positive mindset and improved well-being.

Health Benefits: Planking offers a wide range of health benefits, including improved core strength, better posture, increased bone density, and enhanced cardiovascular fitness. By incorporating planks into your routine, you'll be taking a proactive step toward better physical health.

Start Anytime, Anywhere: You can start planking right now! There's no need to wait for the perfect moment or equipment. Just find a comfortable space, follow the proper form, and give it a try. You'll be amazed at what you can achieve with consistent practice. Remember to listen to your body, start at your own pace, and gradually increase the intensity. Stay committed, be patient, and celebrate every small achievement along the way. So go ahead, give planking a try, and enjoy the countless benefits it has to offer.

# CHAPTER NINE

## The importance of exercise for overall health and wellbeing

Exercise plays a crucial role in promoting overall health and well-being. Physical Health: Regular exercise helps maintain a healthy weight, reduces the risk of chronic diseases such as heart disease, diabetes, and certain cancers, and improves cardiovascular health. It strengthens muscles, bones, and joints, enhances flexibility, and boosts the immune system.

Mental Health: Exercise has a powerful impact on mental well-being. It reduces symptoms of stress, anxiety, and depression by increasing the production of endorphins, which are natural mood boosters. Physical activity also promotes better sleep, improves cognitive function, and enhances self-esteem and body image.

It enhances the efficiency of the cardiovascular system, increases lung capacity, and improves oxygen and nutrient delivery to the body's tissues. This results in improved endurance and the ability to perform daily activities with greater ease.

Stress Management: Exercise provides a healthy outlet for managing stress. Physical activity helps release tension, reduces the levels of stress hormones like cortisol, and promotes relaxation. It can serve as a form of meditation or mindfulness, allowing individuals to focus their attention on the present moment and alleviate mental strain.

Cognitive Function: Research suggests that exercise can enhance cognitive function, including memory, attention, and creativity. Regular physical activity increases blood flow to the brain, promotes the growth of new brain cells, and stimulates the release of chemicals that support brain health. This can improve productivity, problem-solving abilities, and overall mental performance. Social interaction: Many forms of exercise offer opportunities for social interaction and connection. Whether it's participating in group fitness classes, team sports, or

Simply going for a walk with a friend, exercise can help foster social relationships, reduce feelings of loneliness, and enhance overall social well-being.

Longevity and Quality of Life: Engaging in regular exercise has been linked to increased longevity and a higher quality of life. By maintaining physical fitness, individuals can preserve their independence as they age, reduce the risk of age-related health issues, and enjoy a greater sense of vitality and well-being. Remember, it's important to choose activities that you enjoy and that suit your preferences and abilities. Find ways to incorporate exercise into your daily routine, whether it's through structured workouts, recreational activities, or simply being more active throughout the day. Start small and gradually increase the duration and intensity of your exercise sessions. Consistency is key, and even small amounts of regular exercise can have significant positive effects on your health and well-being.

Listen to your body, respect your limits, and make exercise a lifelong commitment to reap its countless benefits for your overall health and well-being.